HEALING A
HOSPITAL

HEALING A HOSPITAL

THE TURNAROUND AT SOUTHEAST GEORGIA HEALTH SYSTEM

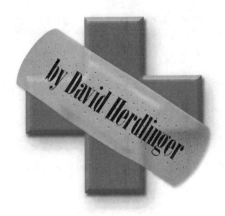

by David Herdlinger

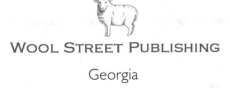

WOOL STREET PUBLISHING

Georgia

Cover Design: Paul Fusch – http://www.macabooart.com

Interior Design and Layout: AuthorSupport.com

Cataloging-in-Publication data is on file with The Library of Congress

ISBN-10: 0-9792325-1-1
ISBN-13: 978-0-9792325-1-0

Published by Wool Street Publishing

This book is available at special quantity discounts to use as
premiums and sales promotions, or for use in corporate training
programs. For additional copies or more information, please contact
Wool Street Publishing
133 Worthing Road
Saint Simons Island, GA 31522
912.634.5777

To William H. Stewart,
a mentor to many

CONTENTS

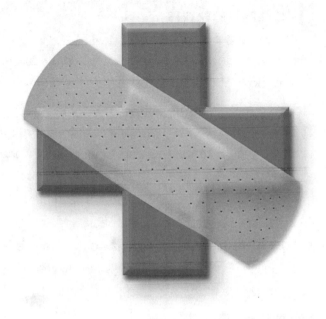

ACKNOWLEDGEMENTS

I owe a tremendous debt of gratitude to so many people who have championed this book into existence.

The fine men and women of Resource Associates Corporation (www.rac-tqi.com) and the Coach Training Alliance (www.coachtrainingalliance.com), and especially Tammy Kohl and Will Craig, have made invaluable contributions, not only to this book, but to my entire career as a coach. Both of these exceptional organizations are setting the pace in the development of new coaches and the preparation of state-of-the-art coaching materials. I am sincerely thankful for their nurturing support and encouragement.

My special, heart-felt appreciation is extended to Gary Colberg, the members of the board of directors, and the other outstanding professionals of the Southeast Georgia Health System. They kindly and generously shared their time and their insightful personal observations so that others can benefit from their wonderful success. This is THEIR story, and I consider it a privilege and an honor to be able to tell it.

The name of my exceptional editor, Michael J. Dowling (www.MichaelJDowling.com), should be on the front of this book. His professional and thorough writing and editing skills were indispensable at every stage of this book's development. Mike edited my first book, *10.5 Reasons Why Even Top-Notch Executives Fail,* and I look forward to working with him on many more projects in the future.

I wanted the cover of this book to be a WOW experience, and Paul Fusch (www.macabooart.com) made that happen. I believe Paul has a magic touch with graphic design, as I'm sure all who touch this book will agree.

Sue Frantz, my outstanding virtual assistant, employed her amazing organizational and clerical skills to virtually pull this book together. She dazzles me with her unparalleled ability to decipher my intentions and develop clarity from my often haphazard thoughts. Everyone who has come in contact with her on this project absolutely loves her, and I am no exception.

To the many friends and colleagues who reviewed drafts and opined on the graphics for this book as it transitioned from concept to reality – thanks!

Most of all, I want to convey my deepest gratitude to my wife, Nancy. With unselfish patience and understanding she endures and supports my demanding career of coaching, speaking, writing, business building, and client management – even as she builds and operates her own high-end women's retail clothing store. It's not easy being Mrs. David Herdlinger, and she excels. Nancy, you're truly a blessing!

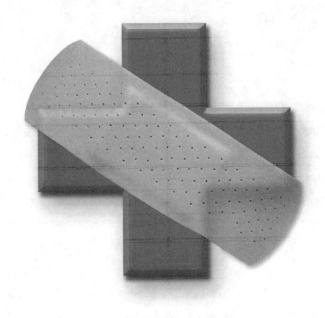

PREFACE

P eople hire coaches out of one of two reasons: inspiration or desperation.

When I entered Delaney's Bistro on St. Simons Island, Georgia, on that late summer day in 2004, I wondered which situation would I encounter. Seated at the table were three key members of the management team of the Southeast Georgia Health System: Tim Chandler, a member of the board of directors, Rachel West, the vice president of human resources, and Gary Colberg, president and CEO.

After some pleasantries, Gary got down to business. "David, I played football in college, and I know the importance of teamwork. I also know the value of good coaching. I want to talk with you about coaching me and some other health system managers. We're making great progress, and I don't want us to be satisfied until we're the best. I think we're going to need coaching to get us to the next level."

There was my answer. Gary wasn't desperate. He was inspired to achieve excellence, and he was assembling the team to make it happen.

It's been my pleasure and privilege to work with Gary and many other talented and dedicated leaders at Southeast Georgia Health System since that day. I've watched an exciting story unfold and have had the satisfaction of playing a modest part.

The story of the Southeast Georgia Health System is too exciting not to be told. That's why I'm writing this book. As I do so, I have three audiences in mind.

First, other communities and their health systems

should find many of the principles and ideas the health system has implemented to be useful and encouraging. Too often we remain isolated from one another and don't make the effort to exchange valuable information. I hope this book helps bridge that gap.

Second, I am convinced that the management principles and techniques Gary espouses and practices will be useful to managers in all types of industries. At a fundamental level, hospitals are businesses. All business managers can benefit from the experiences and successes of the Southeast Georgia Health System.

And finally, I hope this book will be informative and encouraging to our own community here in southeastern Georgia. We all can take pride in the accomplishments of the Southeast Georgia Health System, because every member of the community shares in the success.

Yes, I was hired out of inspiration, not desperation. But before I arrived on the scene, there was indeed a bit of desperation in the air. To paint a more complete picture, we'll begin our story five years earlier.

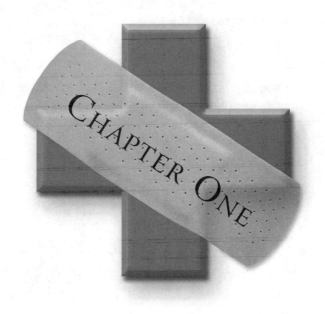

ALARMING SYMPTOMS

Most serious illnesses come on gradually. The first symptoms to appear may be small, hardly notice-able. Over time they become more pronounced and worrisome.

So it was with the Southeast Georgia Health System. In the mid-1990s, the hospital, known then as the

Southeast Georgia Regional Medical Center, appeared healthy. Buoyed in part by cumulative rate increases of 45 percent over the past few years, it was generating sizable profits. The hospital's balance sheet boasted cash and marketable securities of over $60 million, and very little debt.

But during the next three to four years, things began to unravel. Perhaps the management company that ran the hospital was preoccupied with the $60 million facilities expansion project in progress and was devoting insufficient attention to operations. Or perhaps the strong balance sheet and sizable income from investments had fostered a false sense of complacency.

When the stock market plunged in 1998, the hospital's income from investments tumbled sharply. Operational income had already been declining, because over the previous five years management had continued to add employees, while holding rates for services firm. The hospital began to experience a profitability squeeze.

Tensions always exist between the administrative personnel who manage hospitals and the medical staff who use them. The two groups derive their income from the same pool of patient fees, insurance payments, and Medicare reimbursements. To a significant extent, it's a "zero-sum game." Actions by one party to increase its revenues typically diminish the revenues of the other party. The rising influence of HMOs and the corresponding pressures on the healthcare industry to reduce costs added to the strains during this period.

The doctors who practice in the community are crucial customers of the hospital. They have many alternatives if they don't like the services they are receiving. For example, they can choose to take their business to another medical facility. Or they can become competitors of the hospital by duplicating in their own offices some of the services offered by the hospital.

During this heated economic climate, many members of the medical staff cut back their usage of hospital services. As the medical center's cash flow tightened further, management postponed purchases of capital equipment and failed to properly maintain and upgrade existing facilities.

Relationships between the administrative staff and the medical staff deteriorated. The situation hit bottom in the fall of 1999, when the medical staff passed a vote of "no confidence" in the management company that ran the hospital. "It was an awfully unpleasant situation," recalls Dr. Harold Kent, who was chief of staff at the time.

The Southeast Georgia Health System is a state-empowered private entity. A nine-person board of directors, called the Glynn-Brunswick Memorial Hospital Authority, oversees all operations. Since the 1970s, successive boards had chosen to engage the services of professional hospital management firms to run the hospital. The current management firm had been in place since 1989. The hospital's chief executive officer and the chief financial officer were employees of the management company. They had responsibility for all day-to-day operations, including the hiring of the hospital's employees.

As community medical professionals withdrew their support, the hospital's revenues dropped dramatically. Losses from operations ballooned to $1 million per month. Income from investments, which previously had masked the decline in operating profits to some degree, was no longer sufficient to plug the gap.

"At first it wasn't easy to see the full scope of the problems," admitted one member of the board. "The situation was kind of foggy. But we began to feel increasingly uneasy with some of the decisions management was making. And when we started to see the losses, red flags went up."

During this crisis the board met frequently, sometimes

daily. It was not unusual for board members to spend more than twenty hours per week on hospital business, in addition to holding down their own full time jobs.

The pressures were intense. Often the board was divided about what to do.

"Can we ride it out?" they asked themselves. "Should we change management companies? Should we get rid of the management company and take over management of the hospital ourselves?" All were frightening options with enormous risks.

But the risks of doing nothing were even greater. The problems were infecting employee morale and community confidence. Finally, in the late summer of 2000, a consensus emerged. Based in part on the advice and encouragement of local business leaders and physicians, the board voted not to renew the contract with the management company when it expired that October. They decided to look for a president and CEO to run the hospital. The medical center would again be a community-run institution.

"Getting rid of the management company and moving to a locally operated hospital was the biggest, scariest business decision I ever made in my life," one board member told me. "But it made sense because of the upside potential. We're in a growing area that we knew should support a first class medical center."

"Management companies may work fine," said Linda Pinson, a local business leader who currently chairs the board, "if their model fits your community. But the feedback we received from business and community leaders convinced us that our community needed something different."

Brunswick, Georgia, is on the Atlantic coast, about seventy miles south of Savannah, and seventy miles north of Jacksonville, Florida. A five-mile causeway links Brunswick with the beautiful beaches, attractive homes, high quality resorts, and championship golf courses of St. Simons Island and Sea Island. Historic, scenic Jekyll Island is a pleasant fifteen-minute drive south. The region is appropriately called the Golden Isles.

The Southeast Georgia Health System comprises two hospitals and several outpatient centers that serve an eleven-county population of approximately 250,000. The system's flagship 316-bed hospital is in Brunswick. A 40-bed community hospital is located some forty miles south of Brunswick, in St. Mary's, Georgia, the home of the U. S. Navy's East Coast ballistic missile submarine base.

The board notified the management company that its contract would expire on September 30, 2000. That meant the hospital had to have a new CEO in place almost immediately, which of course was impossible. So the management company agreed to send in an interim CEO to continue to operate the hospital. "They weren't legally obligated to do so," explained a member of the board, "but they wanted to help ensure a smooth transition."

"On behalf of the board I contacted Michael Blackburn," said board member Dr. Eric Segerberg. "He had been our CEO a few years earlier when I was chief of staff, and he now headed up a large emergency room physician contract group in Texas. Michael recommended an executive search firm in Atlanta, and gave the search committee valuable advice throughout the hectic transition period."

"It was a smart move engaging the services of that executive search firm to help us find the new CEO," commented a board member. "They specialize in recruiting medical professionals and did an excellent job. As I recall, their fee was $100,000. That's a lot of money, but you have to keep in mind that we were losing that much every three days."

To lay the groundwork for the new CEO, the board decided to swallow two bitter pills. First, they told the interim CEO to lay off 10 percent of the workforce, which over the years had become somewhat bloated.

"We knew there had to be layoffs," a board member recalled, "and we didn't want that unpleasant task to fall to the new CEO. We wanted people to see him as the savior, not the terminator."

"The RIF (reduction in force) was an extremely painful process," confessed one department director. "I had to lay off some really good people who were badly needed. I guess management wanted to appear fair and lay off the same percentage across the board, or maybe there wasn't enough time to look at the decision position-by-position. Whatever the reason, they just told all the department managers to lay off 10 percent of their staffs."

Second, for the first time in five years, the board raised the hospital's rates for services. "These rate increases covered only about 25 percent of our patients," explained a member of the board, "because so many people are on Medicare or other insurance plans that have fixed rates. But it immediately helped reduce the losses to some degree."

When fiscal year 2000 ended on September 30, the hospital reported an operating income loss, before interest income and interest expense, of $9.4 million. That shocked folks who were used to seeing nothing but black ink!

The hospital was sick, and the prescription had been written. The community would again operate the hospital. The nine members of the board turned their attention to the next high priority: hiring a new CEO.

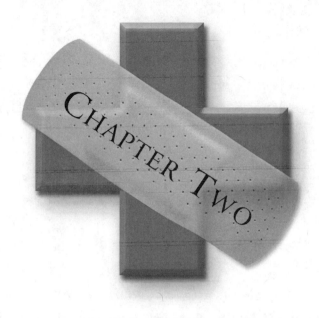

911

On a warm day in January 2001, unseasonably warm
even for south coastal Georgia, an unshaven man
in a T-shirt and shorts entered the front door of the
Southeast Georgia Regional Medical Center in Brunswick.
He reached to take an informational flyer from the "Take
Me" rack, but it was empty.

The visitor walked across the lobby and proceeded down a hallway, entering areas where he should not have been permitted to go. Finally, a nurse approached him. "May I help you?"

"I'm from out of town and I'm contemplating a move to this area," replied the stranger. "Can you tell me what kind of healthcare is available for my family? What's this hospital like?"

The mysterious man was Gary R. Colberg. That morning he had flown into Jacksonville, Florida, from Birmingham, Alabama, rented a car, and driven an hour north to Brunswick. Tomorrow the hospital's board of directors would interview him for the job of president and CEO. Gary regarded interviews as two-way conversations, and he had come a day early to do his homework.

Colberg had not been actively searching for a job. He was satisfied and successful as the senior vice president of Eastern Health System in Birmingham, where he served as the chief executive officer of its flagship 365-bed hospital. But when a leading executive search firm called him about the opportunity in Brunswick, he decided to at least check it out. He had emerged as one of five front-runners from an initial pool of several hundred applicants.

Gary likes to tell people he's from the South. He is…sort of. He's from south Jersey. He graduated from Lycoming College in Williamsport, Pennsylvania, where he played football. After six surgeries on his knees, he decided he'd rather be on the other side of the medical relationship. He entered the healthcare field as a unit manager of a hospital.

Over a ten-year span, Colberg served in two different hospitals in Williamsport, advancing rapidly from unit manager to materials manager to director of primary care to vice president of outpatient care. While working full time, he earned a Masters in Community Health Administration from Vermont College / Norwich University in Montpelier, Vermont.

In 1986, Methodist Evangelical Hospital convinced Gary to move to Louisville, Kentucky, to become vice president of professional services. Within four years he had become the hospital's chief operating officer.

In 1990, Colberg moved to Wheeling, West Virginia, to become the chief operating officer of the Ohio Valley Medical Center. In 1992, he was lured back to Louisville to become the vice president of the Jewish Hospital Health Care System, with its 300-bed flagship hospital. He served there ten years, eventually becoming chief executive officer, before moving to Birmingham in 2000.

Colberg's twenty-five years in healthcare had been busy. So busy, in fact, he didn't even know before the search firm called him that Georgia bordered the Atlantic Ocean. Now, a day before his interview, he was on a steep learning curve.

Over the next couple of hours, Gary asked the same open-ended questions to six other hospital employees. He noted that they frequently began their answers with the words "our hospital." That was encouraging evidence of loyalty.

But, alarmingly, the employees ended virtually every sentence with something negative.

"Our hospital is short staffed."

"Our hospital's equipment isn't up to date and a lot of it doesn't work."

"Our hospital doesn't have enough doctors."

The employees talked freely about the hospital's numerous problems – too freely, considering Colberg was a total stranger.

Later that evening Gary visited two local grocery stores and questioned random shoppers. A picture emerged of a hospital in need of leadership. He had learned from experience that seemingly little things, such as empty literature racks, indicate more significant issues are probably being overlooked. Now his talks with employees and citizens confirmed this. At his interview tomorrow he'd share his observations with the board. Whether they hired him or not, they should know these things.

But he'd also encourage them. He'd tell the board that he thought the medical center had loyal employees and tremendous potential. And he'd commend them for initiating a nationwide search for a new CEO. They were on the right track. They had recognized that they had a medical emergency and they had called 911.

"We interviewed several candidates," recounted board member Tim Chandler, "and Gary clearly emerged as the frontrunner. The whole board came together; the vote was unanimous. We hired him and gave him the authority to do what was needed to turn the hospital around."

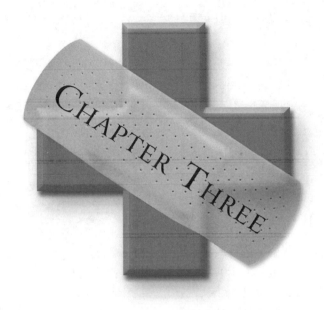

A SOBER DIAGNOSIS

When Gary Colberg reported for duty as president and chief executive officer in late March 2001, morale was poor. A reduction in force the month before had terminated 10 percent of the workforce, representing 132 full-time-equivalent positions. People were angry and discouraged…and scared.

"It was professionally the most frightening time I'd ever experienced," recalled one nurse manager. "Lots of spark went out of people when we had the RIF. We all had lots of questions. The uncertainty was overwhelming."

At 8 a.m. on his first day, Gary convened a meeting of the health center's management team. Eight vice presidents and approximately eighty nervous directors and managers assembled in the Brunswick hospital's conference center to meet their new CEO.

Colberg got right to the point. "I came here to work with you. I want to help you make this hospital the best medical facility in this part of the country. I've played sports; I know the value of teamwork. Every one of you is a valuable member of the team. If we work together, we'll pull ourselves out of the hole we're in and go on to bigger and better things. But we won't achieve success without teamwork. Working together works!"

The atmosphere was tense. Most people were waiting for the other shoe to drop.

"I've had surgeries," continued Gary, "so I know what it's like to be a patient. I want us to look at everything we do from the patient's perspective. Yes, we'll be giving a lot of attention to administration. We're a business, and we need to operate efficiently. But our highest priority is serving our customers. Patients are our customers."

The new CEO proceeded to talk about his agenda and his expectations. "For the next 120 days, I'm going to look, listen, and learn. I want you to be honest with me. If I'm big, fat, and ugly, tell me. I'll do the same with you. I'm a damn Yankee[1]. I like it when you're straight with me, and I'll be straight with you."

"Tell me your problems and concerns," he continued. "But most of all, tell me your 'fixes.' We don't need consultants. You work here, and you know what we should do. I want to hear from you what the solutions should be."

In spite of Gary's enthusiasm, many people were cautious. "Well, we've met the new guy. Let's see how long he lasts."

But others were more optimistic. "It was incredible when Mr. Colberg arrived with his vision for what this place could become," one manager told me. "He told us he was here to help us. He said, 'Let's fix this together.' We didn't know if we could trust him at first. But soon we started moving forward."

"Prior to Gary's arrival," a director remembered, "it felt as if the organization was imploding. Good people

---

1   A Yankee is someone from the North who comes to the South to visit. A damn Yankee is someone from the North who comes to the South to live.

were leaving, and the 'A' players who stayed were frustrated in their jobs because they weren't allowed to grow. When we had the management change, it seemed like a weight had been lifted. To most of us the changing of the guard brought hope."

During the first three months Colberg worked sixteen-hour days. He brought in Michael Browning as the new chief financial officer. In the mid-90s the two had worked together at the Jewish Hospital in Louisville. Sometimes with Michael, sometimes alone, Gary visited every department and talked with every director and manager.

"The first big thing I noticed was how visible the new management was," said a director. "In the past, those of us in middle management interacted with some of the vice presidents and occasionally with the CEO. But the rank and file never saw them. Now, Gary and the other top managers were everywhere."

"Some people were suspicious and a bit paranoid at first," a director commented. "They thought Gary and Michael were looking for 'gotchas.' But over a period of months people realized that they weren't trying to catch people doing wrong. They were trying to spot future stars so they could open up opportunities for them to shine."

Colberg regularly came in at 2 a.m. and walked through every part of the hospital, greeting team members and talking with patients. "Our staff appreciated it," said one nurse manager. "So did the patients. We were impressed that the CEO cared enough to visit the night shift. No member of top management had done that before. We wondered, when does this guy sleep?"

Gary referred to the staff as "team members" rather than "employees." Some saw it as simply semantics. "This hospital doesn't care about its employees," they grumbled, "no matter what they call us."

But others were more positive. "Looking back, it seemed like a small thing," recalls one director, "but actually it made a big difference. When we started calling ourselves team members, it constantly reminded us that we are all in the same boat, rowing forward. It helped us realize that we all needed to work together and that we all had our important parts to play. Cooperation and morale went up."

"My colleagues and I started getting asked to give our opinions about things," said a director. "Sometimes Gary would call us on the phone and ask, 'What do you think about this idea?' But more often he'd just pop in, unannounced. He'd stop team members in the hallway and say, 'How are you?'"

"Before long, people began to talk about how Gary Colberg, the CEO and president, knew their names," remarked a director. "Of course, we had badges and he might have glanced at them sometimes. But regardless, we had a sense that he cared about us as people. That changed the whole atmosphere of this organization. As people began to feel more comfortable, they were more willing to share their ideas and concerns."

One of the first things that Gary learned was that it wasn't easy to find his way around the facility. "I'm geographically challenged," he admits, "and it was three months before I realized that the first digit of the four-digit room number referred to the building, not the floor. And if I was confused, how could we expect visitors to find their way?" He made a note that the hospital's 'way-finding' needed to be more customer-friendly.

As Colberg continued to ask questions, he learned some things that were more disturbing. The RIF that had occurred a month before he arrived had left several vital positions vacant. For example, the hospital now had no diabetic educator to serve the community. In addition, the person in charge of raising money from philanthropic foundations had been laid off. This position typically more

BARB —

I miss you More

You Don'T Fin This

so funny —

than paid for itself, but no one else had been assigned to fill the void.

During the financial crunch of the previous year, management had curtailed investments in equipment. Consequently, much of the equipment was becoming outdated or not working properly. New technologies had not been pursued and necessary additional equipment had not been purchased.

Under Gary's barrage of questions, the "blame game" erupted in full force. But from day one he preached ownership, pride, and teamwork. "This is not about pointing fingers," he reminded the team members, " or what happened in the past. It's about fixing the problems so they don't happen in the future. Remember, when you point a finger at someone else, three fingers point back at you."

The hospital's relationship with the doctors in the community was dismal. Gary paid a "house call" on every member of the medical staff. "Tell me what problems you see and what you need from us," he said over and over in private meetings in their offices.

Meanwhile, Gary set up town hall meetings in the community – at churches, fire stations, and other public locations. The hospital placed ads in the local newspapers, inviting citizens to come to vent their grievances and offer suggestions.

Often eighty to ninety people would show up. "I felt as if I had a target on my chest," recalls Gary. "Aim here. Tell me what you don't like about the hospital. I got killed, but it was the only way to get to the truth."

Colberg took the comments and ideas back to his management staff. Gradually some common themes began to emerge from the interviews with team members, medical staff, and citizens.

For the first 120 days he had listened, learned, and mostly kept silent. The diagnosis was in. The bad news was that the hospital was in critical condition. Gary figured it would take two years just to stabilize the patient.

But there was also good news: the long-term prognosis was favorable. With proper treatment the patient would make a full recovery.

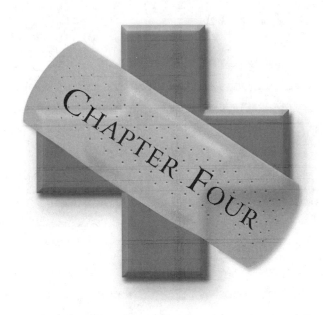

THINKING WELL

G ood morning! Welcome to the team."

Thirty or so eager faces looked up at the speaker from their seats at tables arranged in horseshoe fashion in the hospital's conference room. It was 8 a.m. of their first day on the job.

If the hospital was going to succeed, it needed a new

way of thinking. Colberg's primary goal during the next year was to change the mindset — the culture — of the organization. To help accomplish this, he placed high priority on addressing orientations like this one, held every two weeks for each new group of employees.

After allowing some time for the participants to introduce themselves to each other and to meet the senior management staff of the hospital, Gary launched into his presentation.

"During the next day and a half you'll learn about who we are and how we operate. I'm going to talk about our organization's mission and values. Let's begin with an exercise: When I say a word, you tell me the first word that comes to your mind. OK?"

Heads nodded affirmatively.

"Salt."

"Pepper," answered several people in unison.

"Peanut butter."

"Jelly," came the quick reply.

"Hospital."

A dozen hands went up, followed by rapid-fire answers.

"Sick."

"Pain."

"Expensive."

"Patients."

"Long waits."

"Bad food."

"Doctors."

"Needles."

"Isn't that interesting?" continued Gary. "Do you see how the word 'hospital' conjures up primarily negative images? 'Expensive, pain, sick, needles...' Typically the best thing that people can say about a hospital is that they got out! I don't want us to think of ourselves as a hospital. We are a customer service organization.

"To be more precise," Colberg went on, "we're in the hospitality business. The word 'hospital' comes right out of the word 'hospitality.' In fact, we're just like a hotel. We have a front desk where people check in, we have rooms where people stay overnight, we serve food, and we have a staff that provides services. But there's one significant difference between a hospital and a hotel. How much do you pay for one night in a first class hotel?"

Silence for a moment, then someone answered, "About two hundred dollars."

"Good," replied Gary. "And for that two hundred

dollars, you expect excellent service with a smile, a clean room, and a restaurant that serves delicious food, don't you? That's what we offer, too. Now, tell me, how much do you think it costs to spend one night in our hospital?"

"A thousand dollars?" someone guessed.

"A little low," replied Gary. "The average cost is $1,500. Now, what kind of service would you expect for $1,500?"

"Perfect service!" someone blurted out, prompting scattered chuckles.

"That's right! We want to give people perfect service. We want them to feel special. That's our goal. And we do our best to achieve it. Can we always achieve that goal?"

The participants looked at each other, not knowing quite how to answer.

"No, we can't," continued Gary. "If we're busy, we'll sometimes make mistakes. The only way to completely avoid mistakes is to do nothing. Busy is better than nothing.

"For example, if you're a nurse and you haven't made a medication error, you will. Why? Because you dispense thousands of medications a year. If you're late one time, that's an error.

"You have to take risks to improve. But if you're

overly concerned about being punished, you'll do what you've always done. We don't want to make mistakes. But if you make a mistake and learn from it, that's a good thing. Admit your mistakes; don't try to hide them. Let's be honest with ourselves and with our customers, so we can move on and do better."

The mood in the room relaxed a little. Yes, the expectations were high, but management was more interested in letting people succeed than in letting them go.

"Look at the carpet on this floor," continued Gary. "Do you see any spots on it?"

Heads looked down. Soon the group had identified several spots, mostly small ones.

"Is this rug clean or dirty? Let's take a vote."

Two voted for clean; the rest went with dirty.

"This rug is clean. It was just cleaned this morning. But to most of you it looks dirty. That's what you would tell others about this rug.

"Perception is reality," Colberg informed his attentive audience. "Overflowing trashcans, stains on walls, and dirty baseboards tell people something about our organization. Uncleanliness gives the impression of lack of care about care.

"What do you think patients look at most in our

hospital? That's right, the ceilings. If ceiling tiles have stains, or there's a spot inside a ceiling light that looks like a bug, patients and their families will perceive that we have a dirty hospital. That will be reality to them.

"Be careful what you say, especially in front of our customers. If a patient or a patient's family overhears you talking about some other department in the hospital that messed up, what will their perception be? Right! They'll think we make lots of mistakes and that we don't work together as a team. You create the image that the public sees.

"If you're having a bad day at home, leave your problems at the door. If you allow your personal issues to cause you to be short with customers, it reflects unfavorably on the whole organization. Our customers will say, 'The hospital staff – meaning all of us – are rude!'

"Notice that I use the word 'customers' instead of 'patients.' That's because many of the people who use our facility aren't sick, but they're still our customers. Some come to get x-rays; others come to eat in our cafeteria. But patients are our most important customers, right?"

Virtually every head nodded affirmatively.

"Then tell me," continued Gary, "if a patient asks for

more morphine for pain, do you give it to him? No? Why not? Isn't the customer always right?

"The truth is, patients are not our #1 customers. Doctors are. Nothing happens without the doctor's involvement. We can't even serve food to the patient without a doctor's consent.

"Patients are extremely important customers. They're our #1a customers. Their families are important customers, too. They're #1b. In a sense, they're all our #1 customers. But everything starts with the doctors.

"Choice is the buzzword in healthcare. Our hospital is only one of many options available to the doctors who practice here. We need to give doctors such exceptional service that they will choose to use our services.

"You are each other's customers. Nurses are customers of the pharmacy. Doctors are customers of nurses. The X-Ray Department is the customer of the doctors. The Physical Therapy Department is the customer of the Transportation Department. We're all customers of housekeeping and food service and engineering.

"The departments of most hospitals operate as if they're silos. I don't want a 'silo mentality' here. Our internal customer relationships are just as important as our external customer relationships.

"If you have a problem, go to the source. Get it fixed. Don't say, 'Administration did this or said that.' Administration is not a person. Terms like 'we' and 'they' create internal divisions. 'We' and 'they' are 'us.' We're all members of the same team.

"The image we have in our minds of who we are determines what we become and what we achieve. Life's too short for mediocrity. Why aspire to be just average? We want to be the best!"

The participants sat up straighter in their chairs, glanced at each other and smiled. Gary's enthusiasm was contagious.

"Always strive to do more than is expected. If patients ask you for crackers, think about what else you can do for them. If they're not on restricted diets, ask, 'Would you like peanut butter, jelly, or coffee to go with that? Would you like cream and sugar for your coffee? What more can I do for you?'

"When someone asks directions, don't just tell them, take them. Hold their arms as you escort them and talk with them on the way.

"Think about your customers. For example, why shouldn't you microwave popcorn on the floor? Right!

The smell will make many patients sick to their stomachs. Be thoughtful and considerate in everything you do.

"When you're in patients' rooms, talk to them and their families. Make them feel at home; let them know you care. Call them by name. Hospitals are scary places to most people. If they know you know their names, they'll feel safer. They won't be so worried that they'll end up in surgery when they're supposed to go to physical therapy.

"The answer is yes! If patients ask you for something and you're not sure if it's allowed, say, 'Yes, I'll get it for you if your doctor approves, and I'll check with your doctor right away.'

"When you say you'll do something, do it! If our customers can trust you to keep your word about seemingly little things, they'll have more confidence and trust in our whole health system.

"Share your knowledge. I've had patients complain that the nurses kept rubbing something in their ears, but they never took their temperatures. That's because they thought all thermometers were glass tubes with red mercury in them that we stick under their tongues. They didn't know that our high-tech thermometers allow us to take temperatures with one swipe inside the ear. As you serve patients, explain what you are doing and tell them how our modern equipment works.

"Use common terminology that everyone can understand. Lack of understanding breeds confusion which breeds fear. Don't say PET scan; say positron emission tomography scan, and then explain what that means. Can you imagine what some customers think when they hear us talking about PET scans and CAT scans? They'll go home and tell people this hospital treats animals and people!

"When you see something that's broken, fix it right away if you can. Don't wait for someone else to do it. If you see a small tear in the wallpaper, first paste it back and then report it to housekeeping. If you simply report it, that little tear could be a big rip before housekeeping has time to fix it. They might have to repaper a wall instead of repairing a tear.

"My job is to empower you to do your jobs, so I'm going to empower you right now to fix wallpaper when you see a tear." As Colberg passes out glue sticks, the room fills with laughter.

"We're just having fun," admits Gary. "Actually, as you'll soon see, we don't even have much wallpaper in our facility. But my point is serious. I want you to consider yourselves empowered to make the changes that will make us better. We're heading for excellence, and every one of you has an important part to play."

Colberg began to bring his presentation to a close. "During the remainder of this orientation you'll meet most of the other members of the management team, and you'll learn more about our operational procedures. Remember that my door is always open to you. Come to my office with any problem, as long as you bring a solution."

During the coming months and years Gary would repeat these thoughts at every opportunity. Changing the mindset of an organization requires consistent, concentrated effort.

"New team members are surprised that Gary spends almost two hours with them during orientation," one director told me. "We have orientations for new team members every other Monday, so that adds up to a big time commitment. But he considers orientations to be one of his most important tasks. He's the first person new team members meet. They love it, because he gives them a good feel for what we're about, and they get a sense of Gary as a person."

"If you continue to think like you've always thought,

you'll continue to get what you've always got." That favorite quotation of Colberg's hangs on the wall of his office. It was going to be his mantra for the next year, and beyond, as he made changing the culture his highest priority. But other priorities were right behind.

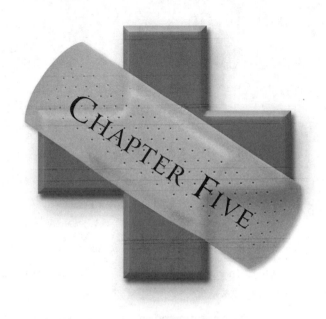

INTENSIVE CARE

The days were long. Colberg typically arrived at 6:30 a.m. and left at 7:30 p.m. He liked to MBWA – manage by walking around – and had a hands-on style.

"No member of top management had ever come to my office," one director told me. "I was shocked to look up from my desk one morning and see Gary and Michael Browning, our new financial vice president, standing there. They had dropped by unannounced to chat with me. In the past if the CEO turned up, it meant I was in trouble. Gary and Mike just sat down and started to chat. They wanted to get to know me personally – what I did in my spare time, if I was married and had children – and to find out how they could help me do my job better."

Changing the culture of any organization requires enormous effort over an extended period of time. People are naturally resistant to change. Settling for mediocrity comes more naturally than shouldering the burdens and risks of pursuing excellence. Pointing fingers is easier than taking ownership. Making excuses is simpler than striving for goals.

The situation at the Southeast Georgia Medical Center was no different. The highway from "hospital" to "hospitality" was not paved.

"I constantly need to remind our team members that we are on the same team," says Gary. "We celebrate our successes together, and we review our failures together. I don't use the word 'problems.' I say 'opportunities.' Our language affects our behaviors and attitudes."

Colberg continued to preach about the importance

of better customer service, and to promote changes that would make it a reality. The medical center instituted valet parking at the front door, so patients and families no longer had to spend time hunting for parking places and hiking from their vehicles.

"Gary got us to stop using acronyms and to speak in understandable English," said a manager. "Now, for example, we say Coronary Care Unit instead of CCU. In fact, it was humorous when we started using the full English words. Many of us on staff realized for the first time that even we hadn't known what some of those initials stood for!"

Customers had trouble finding their way, so the hospital made a long-term commitment to improving "way-finding" by coordinating colors and improving signage. It also changed the names of some departments. For example, people would stand right outside the door of the Health Information Management Department and ask the hospital staff where the Medical Records Department was. Gary changed the name of the Health Information Management Department to the Medical Records Department.

But Colberg ran into resistance when he proposed changing the name of the Imaging Department back to the Radiology Department. "Imaging is the best name," the radiologists argued, "because it's more comprehensive and up-to-date."

"Do you get lost coming to work?" Gary asked.

"No," replied the radiologists.

"Then let's change the name to help our customers who do get lost. The general public doesn't know what imaging means. And besides, if imaging is such a terrific name, why do you call yourselves radiologists instead of 'imaginologists'?"

The radiologists laughed and agreed to the name change.

"It's remarkable what can be done with rather limited funds," one nurse manager observed. "Painting the halls in pleasing, coordinated colors made everything look fresh and clean. The conference room chairs had cloth seats on them that had become dirty. We recovered the chairs in vinyl, and people thought they were new."

Not long after he arrived, Colberg got a call from an irate patient. She complained that she rang her bell for assistance, but the nurse walked right by her door.

"When we investigated," explains Gary, "we found out that the patient had mistaken a member of the house-keeping staff for a nurse. The problem was perception, not service. We changed the nurses' uniforms to royal blue or white, so nurses could be easily identified. Those types of complaints went down to zero."

The new CEO not only preached customer service, he modeled it. On Thanksgiving and Christmas holidays he helped serve meals in the cafeteria.

"Why are you here on a holiday?" some team members asked him.

"Why are you here?" Gary asked in return.

"We're working today," they replied.

"So am I" answered Gary, "and I'm proud to be working along side of you."

When the health center provided a first aid tent at a music festival on Jekyll Island, Colberg helped staff it. "The team members were still cautious around me," he recalls. "But that changed for many when they saw me, dressed in shorts and a polo shirt, serving the public from under that tent in 103 degree heat. That one event, more than anything else up to that time, allowed them to get to know me as a normal guy. After that, they began to trust me more."

Colberg shattered the pre-existing stereotype of a CEO who came in at 9 a.m., sat in his office, and left at 4 p.m. to play golf. For example, on more than one occasion he spent two hours helping the custodial staff move furniture.

At the annual celebrations of Hospital Week, he and the rest of the senior management team grilled hamburgers and hotdogs and served them to the other team members. As distrust of management decreased, dedication and pride increased.

Team members at all levels began to look for ways to provide better service to customers. When they took their suggestions to Gary, more often than not he said do it!

For example, one day a nurse said, "Mr. Colberg, did you know we have metal chairs in the maternity showers? They're rusted and look terrible."

"No," Gary joked, "because I don't shower in the maternity center. But go buy the fiberglass chairs we should have had in there in the first place."

"Really!" she exclaimed. She was surprised, because she had expected to be told there wasn't enough money, or to submit a requisition for consideration.

When another nurse told Colberg that operating room patients didn't like the disposable blankets and pillows the hospital was providing, he switched to non-disposable, high quality items. "We figured it would cost us more," explained Gary. "But you have to spend money to make money, and we wanted to provide first class care. As it turned out, the hospital actually saved money, and customer satisfaction went up!"

"Gary is always looking for the most direct path to excellence," one nurse told me. "One day I noticed he was staring at the floor as he walked down the hall. When he saw me, he said, 'Look at these baseboards. They're all coming loose. I just want to get all the nurses hot glue guns so they can fix them.' We had a good laugh out of it. I could picture all the nurses walking around with glue guns fixing baseboards. But that's the way Gary works. He's even thinking about the fastest way to fix the baseboards."

Does Colberg's passion for excellence sometime cause him to lower the boom too hard? "I saw that happen once," a director admitted, "but in thirty minutes he was back to apologize to that team member. Then he said, 'Let's sit down and have a post mortem on this. Let's look at our options and figure out how we can do it better.'"

To solve the problem of old and dysfunctional equipment, the board approved a phased purchasing approach. Instead of trying to replace large amounts of equipment all at once, the health system scheduled major purchases approximately three years apart. That ensured that some equipment would always be new, some would be three years old, some would be six years old, and the remainder would be ready for replacement.

"We don't hesitate to bring in outside expertise when necessary," one director told me. "When a question arose in the community about whether one of our buildings was sitting on toxic soil, we didn't just try to gloss things over. We hired a professional engineering firm to conduct a study. When we later reported that our facility was safe, we had the data to back that up."

Human resources engaged the services of an independent consulting firm to update job descriptions and make sure salaries were in line with industry standards. They also hired a professional consulting firm to solicit comments and suggestions for improvements from all team members, but participation was disappointing. The trust level was too low to get good results, because in the past management had not respected the confidential nature of such surveys.

Colberg inherited a situation that required significant improvement. I asked a director how he communicates the need for change without being critical and negative.

"Rather than telling people what they did wrong," replied the director, "he prefers to present alternatives. For example, it's been standard procedure for some time for nurses to write their names on a white board in patients' rooms, so patients will know who's caring for them. One day when Gary was visiting with patients on our floor, he noticed in one room that the nurse had not written her name of the white board.

"Most managers would have gone to the nurse manager of the unit and said, 'The nurse's name should have been on the board. Please correct it.' Instead Gary said to the nurse manager, 'If I were the nurse, I'd want my name of the board so the patient would know I'm caring for her.'"

As a business coach, I'm intrigued by Colberg's approach. The two ways of dealing with the issue may seem similar, but actually there's a significant differ-ence. In the first approach, which is more typical, the boss is calling attention to the problem, and telling the team member to fix it. In the second approach, Gary is sharing from his personal experience about how to do something better. He's presenting a vision and giving the team member the opportunity to choose it.

I learned from talking with team members that

Colberg often uses the same approach in assigning tasks. "He's constantly throwing out ideas," said physician services coordinator Mindy Tolle. "Right in the middle of a conversation about something else he may say, 'I've got an idea! What do you think of this?' If you indicate an interest in working on it, he's likely to say, 'That's great. It's your idea. Go for it!'"

To be sure, many subordinates would justifiably interpret the CEO's suggestions as commands. But in fact, Gary has not told them to do anything. He's simply presented visions. Nothing will happen until they choose to accept the challenge. Then they own it; they drive the bus. And Colberg always acknowledges that. He doesn't try to grab the steering wheel. When the project's completed, he gives them 100 percent of the credit.

What happens when Gary presents an idea and the person doesn't pick up on it? "He's a idea factory," continued Mindy, "and he probably doesn't expect every single idea to become a reality. But he doesn't forget anything. If he really thinks it's a good idea, he'll bring it up again at some point. And when you hear it a second time, you'll be wise to give it more attention."

In fact, Mindy's newly created job is one of Colberg's "good" ideas. Reporting directly to the CEO, she serves as the health system's liaison to the medical staff. "I try to make it easier for physicians in the community to work with the hospital," explains Mindy. "I'm particularly interested in discovering problems in the systems and processes. I don't solve them, but I make sure the right people are working on them. For example, right now one of our projects is to make sure the computers in our participating doctors' offices can effectively retrieve information from our medical records system."

Colberg facilitates connections as purposefully as he generates ideas. "In the old days when the management company ran things," said a long-time team member who is now a director, "I rarely got summoned to the CEO's office. If I did, it meant I was in trouble. Gary calls me to his office frequently, and 99 percent of the time he wants to connect me with people and resources that will help me do my job better."

"If something's not going right, Gary wants to know," one director told me. "He doesn't like surprises. But his focus is always on improving patient satisfaction and safety, not blaming. He's got a wealth of experience, and he'll suggest ideas and resources to solve the problem."

Team members responded favorably to the new CEO's leadership. They began working as a team, exhibited more pride in their work, and initiated numerous changes to improve customer service. Surveys conducted by an independent consultant showed that customer satisfaction had increased by 7 percent between 2000 and 2002.

An increase of 7 percent may not sound like much. But in surveys, customers typically rate the very best hospitals only 10 percent better than the worst. An increase of 7 percent meant that within two years the Southeast Georgia Health Center had risen from roughly the bottom third to the top third of all one thousand or so hospitals in the survey.

But changing the culture of the organization wasn't the only concern. The health center needed better administrative and financial systems in order to achieve operational excellence. So Colberg prescribed "fiscal therapy."

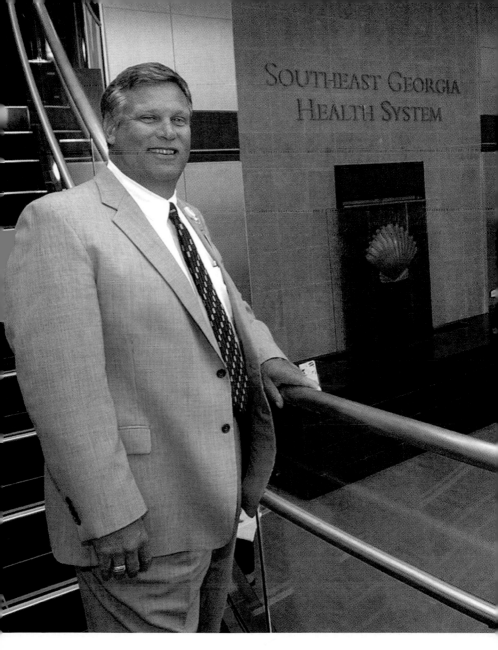

Gary R. Colberg, President and Chief Executive Officer
of the Southeast Georgia Health System

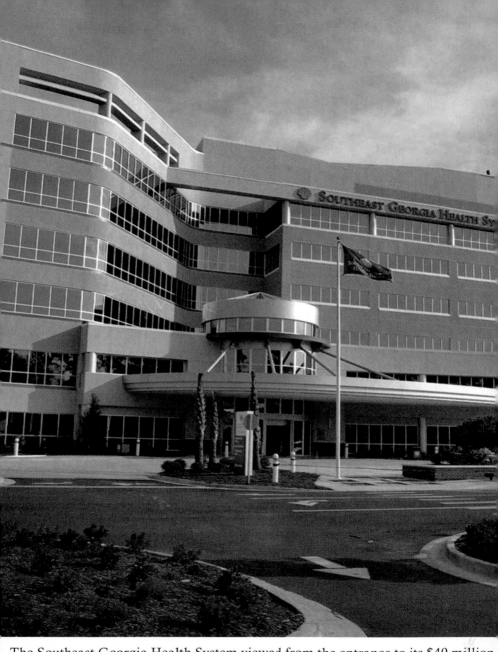

The Southeast Georgia Health System viewed from the entrance to its $40 million outpatient health care and medical office facility, shortly after the new wing opened in April 2006.

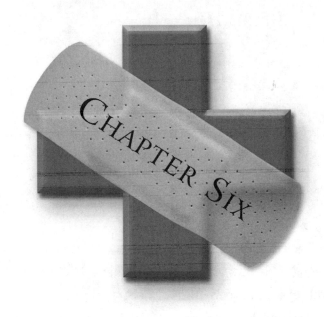

FISCAL THERAPY

F rom the beginning, the new management team went to work to establish the communications, planning, and financial structures that would enable them to successfully manage the business. In order to ensure effective two-way communications, a prerequisite for teamwork, they wove a network of meetings into the fabric of the organization.

Colberg met for two hours every week with his administrative council, composed of the eight or so vice presidents who report to him. They discussed all aspects of the hospital's operations. Between administrative council meetings, he held private meetings for approximately an hour and a half with each member of the council.

Once a month, at noon, the CEO attended a meeting of the board of directors. That same afternoon at three, he presided over a meeting of the hospital's leadership team, composed of the vice presidents and the approximately eighty directors and managers who report to them.

Immediately after the leadership team meeting, the directors and managers met with their direct reports. Thus, information cascaded down from the board to the individual team members on the floors within one twenty-four-hour period.

During the two-hour monthly leadership team meetings, the vice presidents, directors, and managers discussed operational matters, reviewed capital expenditure requests, and personally welcomed all new team members. They also recognized the outstanding professional and personal accomplishments of team members throughout the organization. For example, when operating room assistant Nate Pasco earned a high school diploma at age fifty-six, the leaders honored his accomplishment with a plaque and a standing ovation.

"I had tears in my eyes when the team members at the hospital honored me that way," recalled Nate. "I quit school with a D average when I was thirteen. All my life I'd felt like a failure. When my young son asked if I had finished school, I was embarrassed and didn't want to set a bad example for him. So I enrolled in a correspondence course to get my high school degree."

Nate earned a four-year high school degree in two and a half years with an A average. But it wasn't easy. He had a full-time job at the hospital and a wife and five children at home. During that time his house burned down, his wife was admitted to the emergency room, and his sister almost died.

"Sometimes I felt like quitting," he admits, "but I read in the Bible that trials develop perseverance and faith, and I kept going. When I got my degree, my family gave me a celebration dinner. Mr. Colberg and his wife came, and so did Debbie Hickman, my director here at the hospital. It was a wonderful time. I think my son was proud of me."

The last agenda item in every monthly leadership team meeting is "rumors." "It's a lot of fun," a director told me, "when Gary asks, has anyone heard any rumors? People laugh and start making up rumors to poke fun at each other. But then some real rumors always surface and we set the record straight. That takes the energy out of them, so there's much less gossip in the halls."

Meetings start when scheduled, whether or not everyone is present. "Punctuality is a way of showing respect for others," Gary reminded team members. "Our whole business is built on respect. If we don't respect each other by being on time, how can we expect to serve our customers with the respect and courtesy they deserve?"

At the end of March, the health center reported an operating loss for the first six months of fiscal year 2001 of $3.8 million. That brought the operating loss for the prior twelve-month period (April 1, 2000, through March 31, 2001) to a painful $13.5 million! Chief financial officer Mike Browning immediately went to work to stop the bleeding.

With the assistance of an outside consulting firm, the hospital conducted a "charge master" review of all of fees for services. Some were out of line. For example, in several instances the hospital was charging less than Medicare allowed. The board increased prices where needed.

Concurrently, Browning put high priority on collecting outstanding accounts receivable. He and his team discovered that hundreds of thousands of dollars of bills were uncollected because Medicare had denied the charges. They accelerated the efforts to correct the paperwork to conform to Medicare specifications, so the hospital could collect these funds.

Mike put one director in charge of streamlining the revenue cycle. She and her team made changes throughout the system, starting with the procedures on the floors where charges were entered, proceeding through medical records where the charges were coded, and concluding with billing and collection. All billings, including Medicare, began to flow smoothly from input through collection. Denials from Medicare decreased significantly.

Within six months the hospital had reduced the revenue cycle – the average time from the performance of the medical service to the collection of the billing for that service – from 82 days to 78 days. This freed up approximately $1.5 million for operational purposes.

The health system already had an accurate accounting system, but the management financial reporting left much to be desired. For example, the income statements combined income from operations with income from investments. In the mid-to-late 1990s, the sizable income from investments had obscured the decline in operational performance. Browning reconfigured the reporting so management could clearly distinguish operational income from investment income.

Departmental expenses were out of control. Budgets existed for all departments, but they were imposed from the top down and managers weren't held accountable for living within them. Browning made each department manager responsible for submitting a budget for approval and abiding by it.

Everyone had access to the organization's plan; there were no secrets. Managers were expected to have departmental plans that related to the overall plan. "Plan your work, work your plan, and then celebrate your plan when it's completed," Colberg repeatedly exhorted.

For the fiscal year ended September 30, 2001, the hospital reported operating income of approximately $75,000. That meant that operating income during the most recent six months of the year, since the change in management, had slightly more than offset the losses of $3.8 million for the first six months.

Management awarded 3 percent raises to all team members, plus a cost of living adjustment. "That was my first raise in three years," one director exclaimed. "You can imagine how that lifted my spirits!"

Gary and his team installed a new business planning system for fiscal year 2002, beginning October 1, 2001. He asked all directors and managers to set departmental goals, and to help set the overall goals for the health system. Every goal needed to specify the expected date (quarter) of completion and the name of the "champion" responsible for successful accomplishment.

At the end of the first six months of fiscal year 2002, ended March 31, the health center announced that income from operations was $7.3 million. That brought the total operating income for the most recent twelve months to $11.1 million.

The operating *loss* for the prior twelve months had been $13.5 million. In the year after the arrival of new management, the health system had experienced an operating income turnaround of more than $24 million!

In May 2002, all team members received another 3 percent pay increase, and team members in some positions received an additional market adjustment. Morale continued to climb.

After a three-month study of the available alternatives, the health system in the fall of 2002 purchased and installed a new computer system that better suited its needs for cost accounting, product line management, budgeting, and variance reporting.

Browning began conducting "Finance 101" classes once a month for all members of the leadership team. The classes, which continued for a full year, taught managers how to read financial statements, prepare budgets, control expenses, and write business plans. The hospital unleashed the entrepreneurial spirit by inviting every team leader to propose new revenue-generating business lines.

Colberg set up numerous task forces and workgroups to think strategically about specific issues. For example, he charged a task force composed of team members from various departments and levels with responsibility for looking at operations from an interdisciplinary, multi-facility perspective. Their goal was to ensure that systems and procedures throughout the medical system were smoothly integrated and consistently applied.

"Task forces have been an extremely important

vehicle for improving our operations," one director told me. "When we're asked to serve on a task force, we consider it an important aspect of our regular job assignments, not a diversion."

For fiscal year 2002, ended September 30, the health system reported operating income of $15.4 million, a healthy increase from the $75,000 figure for the prior year. Other indicators were also going in the right direction:

⊚ Revenues year-to-year had increased by 14.5 percent.

⊚ The operating margin, which measures operating income as a percentage of total operating revenues, had increased from a negative figure to a positive 7.6 percent. That was well ahead of the national average of 3 percent for all community hospitals.

⊚ Days of cash on hand had increased from 131 to 167. The generally accepted standard for strong hospitals is 185 days of cash on hand, which means that the hospital could operate for that period of time without additional income.

Colberg had thought it would take two years just to stabilize the patient. Things had progressed faster than he had anticipated because team members had pulled together. In an atmosphere that welcomed innovation and applauded excellence, creative ideas had bubbled to the top and initiative had flourished.

"I couldn't have possibly come into this new situation and orchestrated such rapid change from the top down," Gary acknowledged. "I was still struggling to find my way around the buildings. The staff did it. I simply pointed them in the right direction and empowered them."

When the medical center's independent financial accountants conducted their annual audit, they were overwhelmed by the magnitude and speed of the turn-around. "Come speak at our annual national conference in Charleston, South Carolina," they pleaded. "Our other clients, especially hospitals that are in dire straits, need to hear what you and your team have accomplished."

The following May, Colberg and Browning told their story to over 2000 senior managers from all over the southeastern United States. Appropriately, Gary entitled the presentation, "What a difference a year makes!"

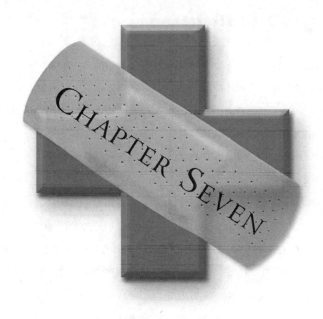

A RAPID RECOVERY

I ntensive Care had ended, but the intensity continued. Colberg's mantra now seemed to be a favorite quote of his by Abraham Lincoln: "Things may come to those who wait, but only those things left by those who hustle."

Quarterly Gary held "CEO meetings" to personally

update all team members on new developments and answer their questions. In order to make it possible for every team member in the organization to attend, he scheduled approximately ten meetings at different facility locations over the course of three days and nights. Team members appreciated this exposure to the CEO. These meetings gave Colberg another forum to talk about the importance of pride, ownership, and customer service.

Also quarterly, the entire leadership team spent a full day reviewing goals and plans. "Some organizations call these offsite gatherings 'retreats,'" says Gary, "but we call them 'advances.' We're going forward, not backward."

Management uses advances as another opportunity to thank the leadership team for their hard work. The meetings typically take place in pleasant settings, such as first class hotels with ocean views. The agenda includes a delicious luncheon and a social gathering at the end of the day. "We work hard, and we also have fun," observed one director.

"When you have an idea or need, think from a system perspective," Colberg reminded his leadership team. "Don't just think about your own department. Call other departments to see if they have similar concerns. When we think as a system instead of a bunch of silos, we'll benefit from economies of scale and system-wide efficiencies, and the additional communications will help us work better as a team."

When one department submitted a capital expenditure request for blood pressure cuffs, Gary asked at the next monthly leadership team meeting if any other departments needed the same item. It turns out that they did, and the health center saved money by placing a larger order.

The public relations department revamped and expanded the "Monday Memo" that the medical center distributed weekly to all employees. Previously, they had printed this newsletter on two sides of one sheet and circulated it sometime between Monday and Friday. Understandably, some snickered at the "Monday" misnomer.

Soon all team members were receiving a full color news bulletin of six to twelve pages every Monday, without fail. It included articles on health center activities, community events that the health system sponsored, announcements of foundation grants the hospital had received, progress reports on facilities renovation and construction projects, and tips and helpful information about personal health care. The additional time and money invested in the Monday Memo paid off in increased pride, better teamwork, and reduced rumors.

Working with a new ad agency, the medical center developed the PRIDE campaign – People Really Interested In Delivering Excellence. Print and TV ads featured approximately fifty actual team members from all areas and levels in the organization. Before long the community was buzzing about the happy, professional people who take pride in working at the medical center.

Even preparing the ads was exciting and creative. One evening, at the conclusion of two days of filming twelve TV spots, Gary and several others went out to dinner at a local oyster bar with the video crew and the people from the ad agency. "There were about twenty of us," the director of public relations remembered. "We started talking about how excited our team members were to be in the commercials. Someone suggested, sort of as a joke, that they deserved Academy Awards."

That spark ignited a blaze. A mere six weeks later the hospital staged the "Shelly Awards," so named because of the seashell that serves as the health center's logo. This black tie awards ceremony filled all four hundred seats of the elegant Ritz Theater for the Performing Arts in downtown Brunswick.

In attendance were all fifty actors and their families, the advertising and filming crews, and the entire leadership team of the medical center and their families. An exquisite shell ice sculpture graced the lobby of the theater. A large billboard showing one of the ads formed the backdrop for the stage; music filled the theater's luxurious space.

Colberg and Browning opened the limousine doors as the "celebrities" arrived at the theater. The same limousine kept going around the block to the parking lot behind the theater to pick up new passengers.

As the celebrities stepped out of the limousines onto a red carpet, flash bulbs popped. A "network news TV anchor woman" rushed over to the "stars" with a microphone and asked who designed their gowns, what their next picture would be, and other tongue-in-cheek questions.

It wasn't practical to leave handprint impressions in the cement sidewalk, as the movie stars do at Grauman's Chinese Theater. But before heading inside, all the celebrities signed their autographs and made tempera ink handprints on large poster board stars. A closed circuit TV camera chronicled the arrivals and projected them onto two screens inside the theater for all to see.

The audience viewed all twelve commercials that evening. As the "stars" received Shelly Awards for their outstanding performances, gales of laughter erupted at the humorous award categories, such as "best supporting actor in a radiology role."

The excitement of the Shelly Awards reverberated for months. The medical center showed a video of the evening on numerous occasions throughout the organization. The public relations department added photos of the "celebrities" to the autographed poster board stars and placed them along with the print ads on the walls of the hospital's dining room. Team members bragged about working with "real movie stars."

The PRIDE campaign had worked. It had increased pride inside the organization as well as throughout the community.

In March 2003, Howard Sepp joined the team as the vice president/administrator of the health center's 40-bed hospital in St. Mary's (Camden County), Georgia. The Brunswick hospital had acquired the St. Mary's operation around 1982, but it had never received the attention it needed and deserved. Gary had gained confidence in Howard's leadership skills when they had worked together in the 1980s at a hospital in Pennsylvania.

Sepp walked into a hornet's nest. Some disgruntled doctors in the community were pushing the Southeast Georgia Regional Medical Center in Brunswick to sell the St. Mary's hospital to a for-profit health organization. The conflict had spilled over into the press; public hearings were in progress.

"We adopted a systems approach," said Howard. "The Southeast Georgia Regional Medical Center became the Southeast Georgia Health System, and the St. Mary's facility became the Camden Campus of the system. Normally a 40-bed hospital would have trouble surviving in today's healthcare climate. But because we integrated it into our overall operations, we were able to draw on the purchasing power and the expertise of the entire system. Over time we upgraded the facilities and equipment, attracted an excellent medical staff, and offered outstanding service to that community."

The health system installed a new management incentive plan for fiscal year 2003, which began on October 1, 2002. Managers were eligible to earn bonuses of up to 10 percent of their annual salaries, based on how effectively the health system achieved its system-wide goals and how well managers met their personal departmental goals. Directors could earn bonuses of up to 15 percent, and vice presidents could earn bonuses of up to 20 percent.

The following four performance benchmarks are a key part of the incentive plan every year:

◉ Net Operating Margin

◉ Personnel Cost as a Percentage of Net Revenue

◉ Supply Costs as a Percentage of Net Revenue

◉ Patient Satisfaction

The system-wide operational improvement goals in the plan vary from year to year, depending on the needs and priorities at the time. There are usually about fifty of them, along the lines of the following examples:

◉ Develop and implement a system-wide way-finding system.

◉ Centralize the patient transport system.

◉ Establish new service lines to expand patient care and generate additional revenues.[1]

◉ Recruit skilled physicians to enable the medical system to provide a more comprehensive mix of expert care.[1]

---

1   The actual goals for each year state specific quantities so that accomplishment is achievable and measurable.

One day in the fall of 2003, Teri Conlan, the hospital's director of volunteers, came to the CEO's office. "Good news, Gary! We've just won an award from the Georgia Volunteers Association. You need to go to Savannah to receive it."

"You don't need me," replied Gary. "You did all the work, Teri, and you deserve the credit. You go and accept the award."

"But the pink ladies and other hospital volunteers will be so disappointed if you're not there," pleaded Teri. "Don't let them down."

Why am I always a sucker for guilt trips? thought Gary, as he drove to Savannah a few weeks later for the awards ceremony. Walking into the hotel ballroom, packed with 5000 people, he was surprised to see his wife and members of the health system's leadership team already there. He was even more surprised a short time later when he was called up on stage to receive the association's award as CEO of the Year for the state of Georgia!

The Southeast Georgia Health System reported operating income for the fiscal year ended September 30, 2003, of $17.4 million, an increase of almost 13 percent over the prior year. And this had been accomplished while adding 136 new full-time-equivalent positions, completely offsetting the layoffs of early 2001.

"Of course, we didn't necessarily rehire the same people," explains Gary. "Based on the recommendations of the human resources consultant, we created some new positions to better match our needs, and we eliminated a few positions. Also, we moved some people to different seats on the bus, and others got off the bus because they weren't willing or able to meet the higher expectations."

"Gary likes analogies about busses and boats," one director said with a smile. "Sometimes when one of us asks him a question about an area of operations he's delegated to someone else, he answers, 'I'm not Julie. Julie on that project is so-and-so.' Julie is the tour director on the TV program *Love Boat*. It's Gary's way of saying that he wants to stay out of the way and let people do their jobs."

Morale continued to rise. At Christmas 2003, approximately 1,200 eligible full time team members received a nice thank you note from the CEO that included two one-hundred-dollar bills.

Members of the leadership team also appreciated the bonuses they received under the new management incentive plan. "I was speechless when I opened the envelope with my first bonus in it," a director confided to me. "It was a lot, I mean a lot, of money! I can't tell you how helpful it was to me and my family."

As news of the turnaround at the Southeast Georgia Health System spread, a hospital in another state made Michael Browning an offer he couldn't refuse. "Mike had done a superior job as our chief financial officer," says Gary, "and we hated to lose him. But I had to agree, the opportunity was simply too good to pass up."

In December 2003, one Michael replaced another. Michael Scherneck, who had worked with both Gary and Howard Sepp at a hospital in Pennsylvania twenty years earlier, became the new chief financial officer.

"When I arrived," Scherneck related to me, "strongly motivated, well directed managers were already in place. Credibility and trust with the medical staff had been re-established. Facilities and equipment were being upgraded and maintained. I had the privilege of joining a team that was already going in the right direction."

But there was still plenty of work to do. "It's easy to engineer a turnaround," Gary cautioned his leadership team. "The hard part is sustaining it."

Colberg continued to hold town hall meetings to

solicit complaints and suggestions from residents in the areas the health system served. But attendance dropped off, because fewer people had complaints. In 2003 an average of about twenty-five people attended the forums, compared with the prior year's average attendance of ninety. The following year average attendance would drop below ten.

At the end of fiscal year 2004, the health system again reported healthy profits. Operating income before interest income and expense was $13.6 million.

The rapid recovery attracted attention. That same month, the Georgia Alliance of Community Hospitals named the Brunswick Campus of the Southeast Georgia Health System the "Best Large Hospital." Among all the hospitals with over 300 beds in the state, it was the "best of the best."

A SECOND OPINION

A s I mentioned in the Preface, people who hire coaches are motivated by either inspiration or desperation. When Gary Colberg brought me on board as coach in late summer 2004, he clearly wasn't desperate. On the contrary, he was inspired to make the Southeast Georgia Health System the best it could be. I'm grateful for the opportunity to participate in the achievement of that vision.

To fit in with the medical theme, I've entitled this chapter "A Second Opinion." But actually that's a bit misleading. As a coach, I don't give my opinions. My job is to help my clients discover the answers that already reside within them.

A lot of people try to misuse coaches. They want to treat coaches like consultants. I'm not saying one is better than the other; they're just different.

Consultants typically focus on maximizing profitability. Coaches focus on maximizing potential.

Consultants help their clients succeed in their jobs. Coaches help their clients succeed in their lives.

Consultants aim to give their clients answers. They say, "I have expertise that you don't have. I'll tell you what's wrong with your business and how to fix it."

Coaches, on the other hand, do not profess to be smarter than their clients. Rather, they say, "You already have the knowledge to be more successful than you are. But it's not knowledge that's important; it's applied knowledge. I can help you use more of what you already have."

Organizations too often make the mistake of hiring

coaches to shore up the low performers. But Gary knew that kind of "band aid" approach wouldn't achieve his objectives. He asked me to coach his entire leadership team – all of the vice presidents, directors, and managers – totaling approximately 85 individuals. His goal was to strengthen every manager. He wanted to help make the low performers better, the middle performers better, and the high performers better.

Gary anticipated other benefits from the corporate coaching program. He wanted to use it to develop succession planning so the medical center could promote from within. He also saw it as a way to help the members of his leadership team see for themselves whether they were in the positions that were compatible with their goals and that best suited their skills, interests, and temperaments.

Gary had a hunch that through coaching some managers would come to the conclusion that they were in the wrong seats on the bus. Perhaps they had been promoted into positions that had turned out to be too stressful, or that demanded time they'd prefer to spend with their families. These individuals, benefiting from insights gained through coaching, could request transfers to other positions in the health system where they would find greater fulfillment.

Additionally, we anticipated that some managers might become aware through coaching that they were not only in the wrong seats on the bus, but they were on the wrong bus. They would then be in a position to choose to leave the organization to pursue work in other fields or in other healthcare settings.

Although Gary foresaw that coaching might precipitate some disruptive changes in the short run, he wisely perceived that the long-term benefits of having motivated people in positions that matched their skills and interests more than offset any short-term risks and inconveniences.

We decided to first conduct a pilot program with seventeen leaders from various levels within the organization. That would allow us to smooth out some of the logistical wrinkles that are involved with coaching people who work on different shifts in different geographic locations, before extending the coaching opportunity to the other members of the leadership team.

Together we designed a coaching process with three phases. In the first phase, I led seventeen participants through eight group sessions over the course of eight weeks. The sessions provided useful information about communications and leadership. But just as importantly, they established the connection and trust that would be so essential to the success of phases two and three.

"I enjoyed the sessions," one director confided to me afterwards. "They taught me some useful skills. And they made me think about my life and my career – where I was, and where I was going."

During phase two, I conducted three private coaching sessions by phone with each of the seventeen participants. They valued the opportunity to express personal fears, questions, and ideas with the assurance that they would be respected and kept confidential. Although phase two was shorter than phase one, many saw it as even more valuable.

"I appreciated Gary making coaching available to us," said a nurse manager. "No matter how much we like and trust the people around us, there are always things we keep to ourselves. We don't want to burden others because they have their own problems. Having someone I could talk with on a confidential basis helped me sort through some thorny issues."

In phase three, the health system offered the participants the opportunity to continue their personal coaching by phone for as long as they wished. Because Gary so strongly believed in the value of coaching, he arranged for the health system to offer the on-going individual coaching to leaders as a fully-funded benefit.

The on-going personal coaching typically entailed one scheduled thirty-minute phone call per week. But participating team members are free to call me whenever they have a decision or concern they want to discuss. Often our coaching sessions simply help them confirm actions they had planned to take. But not infrequently participants become aware of issues and options they hadn't considered, and they decide to change course.

Immediately following the successful pilot program, I led the entire senior management group, consisting of the CEO and all eight vice presidents, through the eleven-week process. Gary felt it was important for him to set the example in terms of commitment. When a conflict caused him to miss one scheduled session, he made it up.

I then conducted additional coaching programs for the rest of the leadership team, in groups of eight to fifteen. We conducted programs three times a year, one program in each quarter except the fourth. Gary, or the vice president of human resources, Rachel West, always introduced me to the new groups at the beginning of their first session. Because they and all of the other vice presidents had completed the coaching program and endorsed it, the managers and directors in the subsequent groups bought into it with enthusiasm.

Many members of the leadership team at all levels elected to continue with the phase-three individual coaching. "My access to you as my personal coach really helped me navigate through a stressful work situation," a director told me recently. "I knew I could talk with you in confidence and that you would be objective and detached. You challenged me to look at some things differently, and your questions helped me to see for myself what I needed to do. I'm sure I wouldn't have handled some difficult situations as well without your help."

Because of my unique position as a coach to leaders at all levels, I often am able to serve as a catalyst for the "cross-pollination" of useful information. For example, sometimes I have knowledge about people or situations that may be blind spots to the individuals I am coaching. During individual coaching sessions, without breaking confidentiality, I may use questions to help these individuals see issues from different perspectives, so they can formulate the most appropriate actions. To a large degree, that's how I was helpful to the director quoted above.

I am also able to help promote teamwork, trust, and morale by passing on compliments, when given permission to do so. For example, when a vice president told me he was very pleased with the performance of a manager, I said, "I'm coaching that person later this week. May I relay your compliment to her?" He enthusiastically said yes.

In a similar way, I sometimes can defuse potentially troublesome issues. For example, a manager told me during a coaching session about a concern she had with a new administrative system. Because of the organizational structure, it would have been difficult for her to address this concern directly. So I asked, "Would you mind if I alert the leader responsible for that area that some people have expressed concerns?" She readily agreed, and the leader was able to address the concerns before they became problems.

In order for corporate coaching to work, every member of the leadership team must have a high degree of confidence that I will not violate confidences or promote anyone's agenda, including my own. Much of the foundation for this level of trust was laid in the initial eight sessions of the coaching program, when I first connected with the participants. But I am constantly aware of the need to continue to build that connected-ness and trust. If I ever betray a confidence or violate anyone's trust, my credibility and usefulness as a coach to the organization would instantly cease.

Understandably, some organizations would be reluctant to give a coach the freedom and access I have been granted. No matter how trustworthy and profes-sional the coach is, it's natural for the CEO and other senior executives to be somewhat nervous about allowing an "outsider" to serve as a "change agent" to the entire leadership team on a continuing, confidential basis.

The Southeast Georgia Health System's commit-ment to this corporate coaching program is evidence of organizational health. Healthy organizations welcome openness and change because they're focused on achieving excellence. Unhealthy organizations tend to foster secrecy, protectiveness, and fear.

Self-assured CEOs give people the freedom to be the best they can be. Executives who lack confidence tend to feel threatened and attempt to control.

Some people ask me how I handle negative gossip if it occurs during private coaching sessions. For example, what if team members criticize fellow workers, or even their superiors? Don't confidential coaching sessions tempt people to engage in this type of gossip?

Actually, the opposite is true. At its core, coaching is about helping people take personal responsibility for their lives. If clients attempt to engage in criticism, gossip, or blame-shifting during coaching sessions, I encourage them to take a step back. I ask them questions such as, "Are you taking personal responsibility in this situation? Do you think your comments are helpful or hurtful? If the roles were reversed, how would you want this situation handled?"

Coaching promotes teamwork and professional excellence by cultivating personal responsibility. When people accept responsibility, gossip and finger pointing disappear.

As a result of the coaching process, some leaders did indeed ask to be transferred to less demanding positions within the organization. Other leaders over time assumed greater responsibilities. A few leaders self-selected themselves out of the organization. The great majority of those involved in coaching simply became more successful in the positions they already held. In all instances of which I am aware, both the individuals and the organization benefited.

"Coaching helps us focus on important issues and how to resolve them," acknowledged Howard Sepp, vice president/administrator of the health system's Camden Campus. "It's another tool in a manager's toolbox. Unlike some management training programs, it's practical. Coaching has helped me balance my personal life and my professional life. I think it's been a significant benefit to managers who take it seriously."

"The money we have spent on the coaching program has been and continues to be one of our best investments," Mike Scherneck, executive vice president and chief financial officer, testified recently. "Virtually all the people we hire have had training in their specialties, but very few have benefited from training in management. A big part of every team leader's job is making decisions and dealing with people. Our coaching program fills an extremely vital need."

You can imagine how satisfying it is for me to receive this type of feedback. Nothing pleases a coach more than to see the individuals he coaches succeed.

AN ENCOURAGING PROGNOSIS

The prognosis was encouraging. Patient satisfaction, revenues, net operating income, morale, community support, and other vital signs were positive. But Colberg didn't let up. He continued to come in all hours of the day and night and MBWA.

"He stays close to us in a good way," says a manager.

"Earlier this week he dropped by my office to chat at the end of the day. He shows up here a lot. Because of that, a comfort level has developed where people really like him. There's a line we don't cross because he's the CEO. But he's earned our admiration and respect."

"Some CEOs are highly visible in the beginning," a nurse manager told me, "but then they slack off. Gary is just as visible today as he was in his first six months. He'll appear in the middle of the night and ask the charge nurse to accompany him while he visits some patients. He likes to have the nurse on duty go with him, because that lets the patients know that we're a team and that he has confidence in the staff on the floor. The team members appreciate it."

Colberg personally delivers the paychecks to the vice presidents who report to him. The vice presidents in turn hand deliver paychecks to the directors and managers who report to them, and the directors and managers deliver paychecks to their direct reports. This gives the leadership team an opportunity every two weeks to say 'thank you' to every team member in the organization.

"Gary doesn't miss much," said a director. "A leaky pipe in the ceiling is a really big thing to him. He's got everyone looking up at ceiling tiles. We're learning to look through the patients' eyes. But we don't do it because we're afraid of Gary. We do it because we shouldn't have to wait for him to point it out to us. He has high expectations for us — he wants us to excel — and we tend to rise to meet that level of expectation."

"I'll give you an example of how Gary spots opportunities and casts vision," volunteered one manager. "The unit coordinator on my floor had a sister serving in Iraq. She and a nurse found out who else in our department had relatives in the military, and they put photos and descriptions on our department bulletin board. When Gary saw it during one of his walk around visits, he mentioned that would be a great idea for the whole hospital.

"The unit coordinator and the nurse took the initiative, and the project became their baby. With the help of human resources, soon the whole wall outside the cafeteria was covered with names and photos of the relatives of team members throughout the health system who were serving all over the world. The girls were thrilled to be responsible for a project that brought so much excitement and pride to the whole hospital. Gary invited them to a leadership team meeting and acknowledged their efforts in front of all eighty or so vice presidents, directors, and managers. It stirred up so much excitement the local paper did a story on it."

These days quite a few stories about the health system make the local newspapers. As I was meeting with Gary in his office recently, I noticed nine picture frames stacked on a table near his desk. "Those are articles about our team members we've clipped from the papers over the past two weeks or so," he explained. "We frame them and present them at our leadership team meetings."

These small personal touches mean a great deal to people. They're a big reason why team members take so much pride in their work. In fact, as I conducted interviews for this book, testimonies about Colberg's care for team members kept popping up.

"Just this morning the phone rang," one director told me. "It was Gary. He said, 'Last time I visited your area I talked with a team member – I can't remember her name – but she said she would love to go to a ball game if I ever had any extra tickets. I have some. Do you think she would like them? How can I get in touch with her?'

"You can only imagine how thrilled this medical assistant will be to get the tickets," the director continued. "But she'll be even more thrilled to know that the CEO cares enough to remember her and to take the time to call her. Gary does things like that a lot. It's exciting and touching for me to see him interact with the team members who report to me, and with the patients on the floor. In my mind that's the sign of great leadership."

Colberg doesn't shield himself from unpleasant feedback. When people want to talk with the president about a complaint, he takes the call. If he's not in, he calls them back.

But these days the health system gets more positive feedback than negative. In his office Gary keeps a file of cards and notes he has received from patients, families of patients, and the general public. Many write to tell him how grateful they are for the excellent care they received. Some mention the names of specific nurses and other caregivers who were particularly helpful.

Gary also receives notes from team members telling him how much they appreciate working at Southeast Georgia Health System. Of course, he prizes all of these cards and letters. Sometimes, on particularly tough days, he takes them out and reads them. "This job is demanding," he admits, "and occasionally it's frustrating. But the people make it worth it. That's what motivates me."

"This hospital has changed a lot since I started

working here over forty years ago…a whole lot!" said RN Kathleen Williams. "In the early 60s it had three floors. The first floor was for blacks, and the top two floors were for whites. On the first floor some rooms had four or five beds. When the rooms filled up, black patients didn't go upstairs. We'd put them on beds in the halls.

"We black employees ate in a separate small room off the main dining room. They'd give us our food through a tiny window in the wall. Whites and blacks had separate water fountains. It was a pathetic place.

"Michael Blackburn broke the ice on change thirteen years ago when he was CEO," continued Kathleen. "But the biggest changes have happened since Mr. Colberg has been here. I've never seen a CEO who does so much for the employees. We get good benefits, a $250 gift at Christmas, a $20 coupon for groceries at Thanksgiving, and cash for sick days we don't use. And he's friendly to everyone, never too busy to talk. What you see is what you get.

"There're no black-white issues here now. Last year when my brother died, I didn't have any relatives in town. Friends from work – mostly white – took over my house. They did everything for me. Now a lot of us are taking Spanish lessons, so we can talk with the Hispanic patients and team members better. We're one big family."

When an organization focuses on caring for people and rewards creativity, new opportunities tend to present themselves, often in unexpected places. Brunswick is a major seaport, visited every year by hundreds of ships and tens of thousands of seafarers from all over the world. The International Seafarers' Center provides hospitality and assistance to these men and women who typically spend months far away from their homes.

Shortly after Colberg arrived, the executive director of the center called and asked if the hospital could provide a wheelchair for a member of the crew who was coming in on a ship from the Ukraine. He explained that the sailor wanted to take it home for one of his parents who was a double amputee and had no way to get around.

"I jokingly told the director that wheelchairs in hospitals are like gold at Fort Knox," said Gary. "We know we have them; we just don't know where they are. After some searching, we did find one without footrests that we couldn't use, but that would be perfect for a person without legs. We gave it to the sailor."

In the process of meeting this need, Colberg asked

the director, "What do seafarers do when they're sick?" "Quite frankly, nothing," he replied, "because typically they don't have the time, the money, or the proper credentials to leave the ship to get medical attention."

Colberg saw that as an opportunity. He set up a rapid medical response team consisting of a nurse practitioner and other healthcare workers. Soon ships approaching the port with seafarers in need of medical attention were radioing ahead to the seafarers' center. When the ship arrived, the medical team went on board and provided the necessary care.

The health system also operates a nursing station at the port and provides the services of a doctor. The hospital's pharmacy fills prescriptions. "As far as I know, we're the only hospital in the world that provides this kind of service," said Gary. "Now ships are going out of their way to use our port. We have the privilege of serving people from all over the world and spreading international goodwill. And the merchants of our community benefit, because we have more ships bringing more crew members to spend money in our local economy."

Sometimes the new ideas of team members benefit people far beyond the health system's normal region of service. RJ Fernandez, a surgical technician, envisioned ways to improve the bariatric surgical drapes that cover patients during surgery. He shared his concepts with fellow workers, who added their own suggestions. Then he shared them with a representative from Kimberly Clark, one of the health system's major vendors. Today Kimberly Clark markets nationwide a newly designed bariatric surgical patient drape that incorporates innovations conceived at the Southeast Georgia Health System.

Naturally, the leadership team acknowledged RJ's accomplishment at one of its monthly leadership meetings. But RJ isn't the only one in his family who has received acknowledgment recently. When his grandmother retired after fifty years of service, management acknowledged her outstanding service at the annual awards banquet. But that wasn't all. They also drove her to the banquet in a limousine!

The Southeast Georgia Health System has developed strategic partnerships with two outstanding medical service providers in Jacksonville, Florida: St. Vincent's Hospital, one of the leading centers for open-heart surgeries in the Southeast, and Brooks Rehabilitation Hospital, a regional leader in rehabilitative care. It also generously funds the nursing education program at

Coastal Georgia Community College in Brunswick, and provides internships for many of the school's nursing degree candidates.

In 2005 Johns Hopkins Medical Center in Baltimore invited the Southeast Georgia Health System to participate in a three-year nationwide trial. "The study will help shape national healthcare policy," Gary enthusiastically told me. "Johns Hopkins wants to demonstrate that regional hospitals without attached open-heart programs can save lives by performing angioplasty and stenting-of-the-heart procedures in partnership with larger hospitals that do provide open-heart care.

"For example," Colberg continued, "if complications develop during an angioplasty or stenting procedure at our facility, we can immediately airlift the patient to St. Vincent's, our strategic partner in Jacksonville, for more specialized attention. Johns Hopkins invited only forty hospitals in the country to partner with them, and we're proud to be included."

In April 2006, the health system opened a 195,000 square foot, six-story, $40 million outpatient health care and medical office facility. It houses the new cancer care center, a women's imaging center, an outpatient surgical center, and a health information center. Timeshare suites are available for use by out-of-town "super-specialists," so local patients no longer have to leave the area for follow-up visits. The modern technology in the cancer center is more advanced than that available in some large cities, including Jacksonville and Savannah.

The hospital has established an art gallery in the new building where the paintings of respected local artists are exhibited. "I want our facility to be a destination of choice, not just of necessity," says Gary. "I'd like to see people come here after church on Sunday to enjoy a delicious, reasonably priced meal in our cafeteria, and then view a high quality art exhibit."

In 1993 the hospital had 140 physicians on its medical staff. By 2006 the number had increased to about 310. "As the hospital system grew and expanded into surrounding counties, we became more active in recruiting," explains Dr. Eric Segerberg, the board's longest serving member. "The quality of our facilities and equipment and the quality of life in the area have allowed us to attract some highly skilled doctors who might otherwise have practiced in Atlanta or any other large metropolitan area."

On September 30, 2006, at the end of the fifth fiscal year since the arrival of new management, the Southeast Georgia Health System could look back and celebrate five consecutive years of black ink. For every one of the past four years operating income had exceeded $13 million.

The balance sheet reported 258 days of cash on hand, a 100 percent increase over the 2000 level. This meant that the health system could continue to operate for 258 days without any additional revenues, which is 73 days more than the accepted benchmark for a strong hospital.

In 2006 the Southeast Georgia Health System received an "A2" rating from Moody's Investor Services and an "A" rating from Standard & Poor's. In a report of hospitals conducted by Moody's that year, only four out of ten earned a rating equal to or better than that assigned to Southeast Georgia Health System.

A survey conducted by independent consulting firm Press Ganey reported very high customer satisfaction scores. Of the approximately one thousand hospitals included in the nationwide survey, the Brunswick campus received a rating above 90 percent for outpatient care, and above 80 percent for inpatient care.

But the Southeast Georgia Health System doesn't intend to spend much time looking back. As it has prospered, the board and operating management have reinvested the profits. The priorities are employees, technology, facilities, and community, in that order.

"One of the things I am most proud of," says Michael Scherneck, CFO, "is that we have continued to increase our investment in facilities. In 2001, we were investing approximately $6 million per year in property, plant and equipment. By 2006, that amount had grown to approximately $25 million. That's about 12 percent of our annual revenues, which is well above the national average of 8 percent.

"Between 2004 and 2006 our net property, plant, and equipment increased by almost $50 million," Scherneck continued. "That's an increase of over 40 percent. We are committed to reinvesting our revenues in state-of-the-art equipment and facilities, so that we can provide the highest quality care, both now and in the future."

When the new management team arrived in 2001, the public relations budget was miniscule. By 2006 it had grown to approximately $1 million. A considerable portion of those funds are earmarked for community charitable causes, such as the American Cancer Society, the American Heart Association, the American Diabetes Association, the American Red Cross, and the Special Olympics. In addition, the health system provides more than $250,000 of funding per year for the public school nurse program, a similar amount to provide trainers for school athletic teams, and substantial funds for other community needs.

The Southeast Georgia Health System also is the lead sponsor of several community events each year. For example, it organizes Relay for Life events in four counties to raise money for the American Cancer Society. It helps organize and run the annual Brunswick Stewbilee, which attracts more than eight thousand people and raises more than $12,000 for the Boys and Girls Clubs. And it annually provides over $30 million dollars in free care to citizens of the community, an increase of 25 percent since 2001.

"We're particularly proud of the Coastal Medical Access Program," said DelRia Tate, vice president of professional services. "The Southeast Georgia Health System helped organize this not-for-profit institution in 2001 to provide free access to healthcare for uninsured and underinsured citizens. The program is a collaborative effort among the health system, local medical professionals, the health department, the community college, and faith-based institutions. We donate over $250,000 per year for its operational expenses, as well as space for clinics in Brunswick and in Camden County."

"In recent years the Southeast Georgia Health System has evolved into one of the most active corporate citizens in our community," said Woody Woodside, president of the Brunswick Golden Isles Chamber of Commerce. "They sponsor and are involved in numerous programs that benefit our citizens. And the pride and enthusiasm of the people who work there affects our whole community in very positive ways."

"When the community took control of the hospital, it definitely was a good decision," says Hank Rowland, city editor of the Brunswick News, the area's major newspaper. "In the past the health system seemed to be spinning its wheels. Now it's really moving forward. Management is not just thinking about serving the community better today; they're planning and investing to provide better healthcare in the future."

In the fall of 2006, the Southeast Georgia Health System purchased a 78-bed convalescent center in St. Mary's. It plans to eventually build a new facility for this center adjoining the 40-bed hospital it already operates there. Combining the two types of medical services under one umbrella promises to significantly improve the quality of care available for the citizens of that community.

Recently the human resources department had an outside consulting firm conduct another confidential survey of team members to solicit their ideas for improve-· ments. The previous survey, conducted about four years before, had yielded very little feedback because team members didn't trust that their answers would be kept confidential. This time participation was much better, and the survey produced a considerable number of useful suggestions.

"The Board has learned that we can trust Gary," one director told me. "If he says something, he has the data to back it up. He doesn't shoot from the hip. Before Gary came on board, we weren't pulling together. Some of us would spend ten to twenty hours a week at the hospital involved in management. Now, we're unified and board meetings are a pleasure. We provide oversight and attend community functions, and we leave the management to the professionals."

"The Southeast Georgia Health System is successful largely because Gary has built a talented management team that shares a common vision," said vice president Howard Sepp. "We have the right people in the right places at the right time. They bring a depth of experience and expertise that is so necessary in the very complex healthcare field. I'm optimistic about the future."

These days the health system is moving into the future at a rapid pace. In fact, as this book was about to go to press, it embarked on a new phase of its development by acquiring Summit Sports Medicine & Orthopaedic Surgery in Brunswick.

The very word "acquire" can conjure up images of disruption and even hostility. But the health system's philosophy is to value and preserve acquired organizations by incorporating them as functioning entities. On April 11, 2007, Summit's entire staff of six physicians, one physician assistant, and over forty support personnel became enthusiastic members of the Southeast Georgia Health System team.

"The acquisition surprised some people in the community," said Carlton DeVooght, the health system's vice president and general counsel. "They considered Summit and the Southeast Georgia Health System to be unlikely partners, because in the past we sometimes competed for market share. But in fact, our new partnership is a synergistic relationship in which the whole is greater than the sum of the parts. Summit has outstanding physicians and an excellent reputation, and the Southeast Georgia Health System possesses the ability to serve patients who have a wide variety of incomes and medical insurance plans. By joining forces, we are able to offer quality orthopedic care to people who couldn't previously afford it."

"During the first five years of our turnaround, we concentrated on fixing things and building our infrastructure," said Michael Scherneck, CFO. "Now we are entering a positive growth phase to position ourselves for the future. The acquisition of Summit is the first step toward building a Center of Excellence, which will approach treatment comprehensively from consultation to surgery to rehabilitation. Top-flight physicians serving in the key specialties are crucial to the achievement of our mission as a health center. I expect that we will make additional strategic acquisitions in the future when that is the best way to expand our capacity to provide quality healthcare to the communities we serve."

Colberg admires the philosophy of Wayne Gretzky, the outstanding National Hockey League player. When a sports writer asked Gretzky the secret of his success, he answered, "I anticipate. I don't want people to pass the puck to me when I'm standing still. I want them to lead me when I'm on the move. Then I go where the puck is going to be."

"That's what I want to help us do," says Gary. "I want us to always be looking to see where healthcare is going to be in five or ten years, and go there."

Yes, the prospects are exciting and the prognosis is good. But where will all this lead?

"I don't know," Gary answers. "But when you wake a sleeping giant, watch out!"

"I'm entering my twentieth year as a nurse," a team member told me, "and I've been at this hospital since 1994. This is the most challenging thing I've ever done. I can't say I love every thing I do every day – some parts are hard and even unpleasant. But I can honestly say I love my job. I work with the most incredible group of people, both my peers and my bosses. I'm very proud of our hospital. It's writing new chapters in its history, and it's so exciting to be part of that."

ABOUT THE AUTHOR

David Herdlinger is a coach. His company, HERDLINGER ASSOCIATES, provides personal and team coaching services to individuals and organizations worldwide. Through the powerful dynamics of coaching, he has helped thousands of executives and professionals at all levels and in all types of organizations unleash their potential and achieve more than they ever dreamed possible.

David challenges people to "be" before they "become." In fact, he experienced the power of this life principle firsthand as he transitioned through careers in law, politics, business, and organizational development on his way to becoming a full-time coach. Now he has the privilege of helping others travel similar journeys toward greater authenticity and accomplishment.

"When individuals discover their potential and identify their purpose," says David, "they begin to align their attitudes, goals, and actions with their deepest motivations. That unleashes a tremendous amount of focused energy, which results in extraordinary success and fulfillment in both their personal and professional lives. As a coach, nothing thrills me more than watching my clients experience success and satisfaction beyond their wildest expectations."

Herdlinger helps his clients balance their personal and professional lives, so the goals and actions in both spheres are compatible and mutually reinforcing. "Many people make the mistake of compartmentalizing their lives," explains David, "and that sets up tensions that hinder success. Individuals maximize their potential when they view life holistically."

David is a leader and foremost authority on one of the most exciting new frontiers of the coaching profession: coaching corporate teams. "Coaching all, or substantially all, of the members of the management team of an organization leverages the positive results of coaching," says David, "both for the organization and for the individuals involved. It significantly enhances teamwork and communications by ensuring that every member of the team is in the right position and going in the right direction."

David holds degrees in communications and law. His prior work experiences include managing partner of a law firm, prosecutor, judge, law school faculty member, special consultant to an attorney general, healthcare business executive, and organizational development consultant. He is also the author of *10.5 Reasons Why Even Top-Notch Executive Fail, And How To Make Sure It Doesn't Happen To You.* David lives with his wife, Nancy, on Saint Simons Island, Georgia.

ABOUT THE COMPANY

Herdlinger Associates provides personal and team coaching services to individuals and organizations in the United States, Canada, Asia, and Europe.

Through the dynamic power of coaching, the firm helps clients

- discover their potential

- identify their purpose

- clarify their goals

- develop their plans

- implement right actions

in order to achieve maximum personal and professional success.

Herdlinger Associates believes that the potential for

success already lies within every individual; it simply must be discovered and unleashed. When individuals move toward authenticity by identifying their purpose and passion, and when they take responsibility for their lives by cultivating attitudes of accountability, they will more naturally tend to choose the right actions that result in extraordinary accomplishment and fulfillment.

David Herdlinger and his associates encourage clients to view their lives holistically, so that all aspects are aligned and mutually compatible. Individuals achieve greatest satisfaction when they balance the profit motives of their professional lives with the values and desires of their personal lives.

By augmenting its powerful coaching processes with the results-proven methodologies of its strategic partner, Resource Associates Corporation, Herdlinger Associates accelerates clients' development of the skills and attitudes necessary for success.

The firm's clients range in size from individuals and very small businesses to corporations with annual sales in excess of $40 billion.